RENAL DIET

Guide To A Specific Eating
Plan Intended To Help And Treat
Kidney Infection

Joy B. Hunt

Table of Contents

CHAPTER1

What is the renal eating routine

The renal eating routine is a specific eating plan intended to help the wellbeing and capability of the kidneys. Commonly endorsed for people have kidney infection or are in danger of creating it. The primary objective of the renal eating regimen is to diminish the responsibility on the kidneys by restricting the admission of specific supplements, like sodium, phosphorus, and potassium. People can help manage their kidney function, prevent further damage, and improve their overall health by following this diet.

Controlling sodium intake is an important part of the renal diet. Inordinate sodium utilization can prompt liquid maintenance and hypertension, which can overburden the kidneys. As a result, renal dieters are advised to steer clear of processed foods, canned goods, and fast food that are high in sodium. Instead, they are encouraged to select whole grains, lean meats, and fresh vegetables.

The management of phosphorus levels is an additional important part of the renal diet. The kidneys can be harmed and kidney disease can progress when blood levels of phosphorus are high. To control phosphorus admission, people are educated to restrict their utilization with respect to dairy items, nuts, seeds, and handled food sources, as these are many times high in phosphorus. All things considered, they ought to zero in on drinking low-phosphorus options, for example, non-dairy milk, new natural products, and vegetables.

The renal diet requires people to watch their potassium intake in addition to sodium and phosphorus. When a person has kidney disease, high potassium levels can cause complications and disrupt the heart's rhythm. As a result, potassium-rich foods like bananas, oranges, tomatoes, and potatoes should be avoided at all costs. All things considered, people are urged to pick low-potassium options, like apples, berries, green beans, and rice. By intently checking their sodium, phosphorus, and potassium consumption, people on the renal eating routine can really uphold their kidney wellbeing and generally speaking prosperity.

A renal eating regimen, otherwise called a kidney-accommodating eating routine, is explicitly intended to assist people with kidney sickness deal with their condition and advance generally kidney wellbeing. It is essential for individuals with kidney disease or compromised kidney function to adhere to diet focus on managing key nutrients such as protein, specific nutritional guidelines to prevent sodium, potassium, further damage, and maintain phosphorus, and overall fluid health intake. These Protein guidelines focus intake on is managing an important key nutrient considerations such as protein, individuals with kidney sodium disease, potassium, and phosphorus. A renal diet refers to a crucial specific for dietary those plan designed as to certain support foods optimal and kidney nutrients can potentially worsen While protein is fundamental for.

CHAPTER2

The management practices of A renal diet

An essential component of managing kidney disease and preserving optimal kidney function is the renal diet. It is intended to lessen the responsibility on the kidneys, forestall further harm, and oversee side effects related with kidney illness. However, why is a renal diet so crucial for people with kidney disease?

Most importantly, a renal eating regimen assists with controlling the levels of specific supplements in the body, like sodium, potassium, and phosphorus. The kidneys struggle to regulate these nutrients when they are not functioning properly, which can result in imbalances and complications. By following a renal eating routine, people can restrict their admission of these supplements and keep them from moving toward risky levels in the body. This can assist in managing symptoms like high blood pressure and fluid retention and preventing further kidney damage.

A renal diet can also assist in the management of other health issues that frequently accompany kidney disease. Diabetes or high cholesterol, for instance, are frequently associated with kidney disease, which can further impair kidney function. A renal diet can help control blood sugar and cholesterol levels and can be tailored to treat these conditions as well. By dealing with these existing together circumstances, people can work on their general wellbeing and diminish the stress on their kidneys.

In conclusion, a renal eating regimen can extraordinarily further develop a singular's personal satisfaction. Kidney illness can cause a scope of side effects, including weakness, sickness, and unfortunate hunger. By following a renal eating regimen, people can limit these side effects and further develop their energy levels and by and large prosperity. A renal diet can also empower patients to actively participate in their treatment and give them a sense of control over their health. This may help them deal with the difficulties of living with kidney disease by improving their mental and emotional health.

In conclusion, a renal diet is essential for people with kidney disease because it helps to control nutrient levels, manage co-existing health conditions, and enhance quality of life. People can support their kidney function, prevent further damage, and effectively manage kidney disease symptoms and complications by following a renal diet. Individuals with kidney disease must collaborate closely with dietitians and healthcare professionals to create a customized renal diet plan that meets their specific requirements and objectives.

A specialized diet plan called a renal diet, also known as a kidney diet, is made to help people with kidney disease manage their condition and prevent further damage to their kidneys. The primary objective of a renal diet is to lessen the burden placed on the kidneys and prevent the accumulation of fluid and waste products in the body. Following certain guidelines to ensure that the diet is suitable for people with kidney disease is one of the key components of a renal diet.

Limiting sodium intake is the first rule of a renal diet. Both high blood pressure and fluid retention, both of which are bad for the kidneys, can be caused by sodium. Avoid fast food, canned soups, and processed foods if you follow a renal diet to reduce your sodium intake. All things being equal, they ought to zero in on devouring, amazing failure sodium food varieties and utilizing spices and flavors to upgrade the kind of their feasts.

Controlling protein intake is another important rule for a renal diet. Protein is fundamental for the body, yet exorbitant utilization can overburden the kidneys. High-quality protein sources like lean meats, fish, eggs, and dairy products should be consumed in moderation by kidney disease patients. Red meat and processed meats, which are high in protein, should also be avoided.

Ultimately, people following a renal eating routine ought to watch their admission of potassium and phosphorus. Both of these minerals can gather in the body and cause difficulties for people with kidney sickness. Avocados, bananas, and other foods high in potassium should be consumed in moderation. In a similar vein, whole grains and dairy products, which contain a lot of phosphorus, should be avoided. Individuals can better manage their kidney disease and maintain optimal kidney health by following these guidelines.

Lastly, a renal diet is a specialized diet plan designed to help people with kidney disease manage their condition. Individuals can control their intake of protein, potassium, and phosphorus, as well as their sodium intake, by adhering to specific guidelines. In order to preserve kidney health and prevent further damage, these guidelines are essential. Individuals with kidney disease should collaborate closely with a healthcare provider or registered dietitian to create a bespoke renal diet plan that addresses their specific nutritional requirements.

The renal eating routine is a particular eating plan that is intended to assist people with kidney sickness deal with their condition and keep up with ideal wellbeing. In order to prevent the buildup of waste products in the body, it focuses on controlling the amount of certain nutrients, like protein, sodium, potassium, and phosphorus.

Overall, excessive protein management is one of the most important health factors and aspects of a renal diet for tissue repair. Intake is this likely to strain the kidneys? since Subsequently, harmed kidneys those may following battle to a renal channel and eliminate side-effects diet are frequently encouraged to restrict productively. their protein to stop the accumulation of consumption. People with lean kidney disease, for example, are frequently advised to limit their intake of high-quality protein from waste sources, such as fish and eggs. However, it is essential to consume high-quality protein sources like dairy products because they contain all essential amino acids and are low in lean meats like fish, poultry, and potassium.

CHAPTER3

What are the meal plans for a renal diet

The development of well-balanced and nutritious meal plans that cater to the particular dietary requirements of people who have kidney disease is an essential component of the renal diet.

Sample meal plans for a renal diet are carefully crafted to ensure that people with kidney disease consume the appropriate quantities of nutrients and avoid those that could harm their kidneys. These feast designs regularly incorporate various food varieties that are low in sodium, potassium, and phosphorus. A breakfast meal plan might include, for instance, oatmeal with fresh berries and apple juice. This gives a decent equilibrium of sugars, fiber, and nutrients, while keeping the degrees of sodium, potassium, and phosphorus under tight restraints.

Lunch and supper dinner plans for a renal eating regimen frequently comprise of lean protein sources, like skinless chicken or fish, matched with various vegetables that are low in potassium and phosphorus, like green beans, cauliflower, or cabbage. Whole grains, such as quinoa or brown rice, which are a good source of fiber and provide essential nutrients without overtaxing the kidneys, are also included in these meal plans. Fruits with low potassium, such as apples or grapes, and snacks with low sodium, such as air-popped popcorn or unsalted nuts, may be suitable for a renal diet.

Generally, test feast plans for a renal eating regimen are intended to furnish people with kidney illness with a fair and nutritious eating routine while dealing with their particular dietary requirements. These feast plans center around controlling the admission of supplements that can be hurtful to the kidneys and advance the utilization of food varieties that help kidney wellbeing. By following a renal eating regimen and sticking to the suggested feast plans, people with kidney sickness can really deal with their condition and further develop their general prosperity.

The job of nourishment in renal wellbeing is pivotal for people with kidney illness. When the kidneys aren't working properly, it's important to make changes to your diet to help them.

The kidneys remove waste and excess fluids from the body. A renal eating regimen is explicitly intended to assist with overseeing kidney illness and forestall further harm to the kidneys.

One vital part of a renal eating routine is controlling the admission of specific supplements, like protein, sodium, potassium, and phosphorus. Although protein is an essential nutrient for the body, excessive protein intake can strain kidneys in people with kidney disease. In this way, it means quite a bit to restrict the utilization of high-protein food varieties and spotlight on getting the perfect proportion of protein from sources that are more straightforward for the kidneys to process.

Electrolytes like sodium, potassium, and phosphorus can have a big effect on how well the kidneys work. High blood pressure and fluid retention, both of which can put additional strain on the kidneys, can result from excessive sodium intake. Potassium and phosphorus, then again, can gather in the blood when the kidneys are not working as expected, prompting irregular characteristics and likely complexities. As a result, a renal diet aims to maintain adequate body nutrition while limiting sodium, potassium, and phosphorus-rich foods.

In conclusion, people with kidney disease need to know how nutrition affects their kidney health. Protein, sodium, potassium, and phosphorus are managed in a renal diet to support kidney function and prevent further damage. Individuals can contribute to the improvement of their kidney health as well as their overall well-being by altering their diet and adhering to the nutritional guidelines for a renal diet.

S and sodium are important because they provide an additional essential nutrient, amino acids, which must be carefully managed to maintain muscle mass, renal health, and overall health.

Diet. Excessive Another sodium consumption fundamental part of a renal can contribute diet to high is circulatory strain controlling and sodium liquid admission maintenance., Sodium is the two of which can regularly found in wors processeden food sources kidney, canned capability. foods, and as a result, condiments. People with kidney disease are advised to limit their sodium intake because too much sodium can cause fluid retention and higher blood pressure. They should also cut back on processed and packaged foods. People are encouraged to consume fewer processed and packaged foods in order to control their sodium intake and are encouraged to use table salt when cooking. as well as Rather keep away from, adding they can salt flavor during their feasts with spices, flavors, cooking or at and other the low table-s.odium options All things being equal,. In addition, utilizing spices, herbs, and other spices, reading food labels, and selecting flavorings can help reduce sodium and improve the flavor of meals without using sodium-free products

In prescribed expansion to protein and sodium, people observing a renal eating regimen rules.

Phosphorus and potassium are two minerals that people with kidney should likewise screen their potassium and phosphorus consumption. Although a wide variety of vegetables and fruits contain potassium, disease must be closely monitored. Bone and heart problems can result from high levels of phosphorus, and heart rhythm problems can result from high potassium levels. Destructive to people with kidney illness. Those on a renal diet should limit or avoid high-phassiumosph foods like bananas, oranges, dairy, tomatoes, products, and potatoes legumes in order to manage their phosphor Sores intake. Similarly, phosphor whole grains Soorus can be found in certain nuts, seeds, dairy, and dairy products. furthermore, Correspondingly, food varieties wealthy in carbonated potassium, drinks like bananas,, and exorbitant admission oranges, tomatoes, and potatoes can add to bone and heart issues. Accordingly, ought to be restricted. It is, people on a renal eating routine are encouraged to vital as far as possible their admission with of a these enlisted food sources too diet.

In conclusion,itian or medical care proficient to following explicit decide the proper healthful rules levels is significant of phosphorus for people on a renal and potassium for a singular's particular necessities.

In conclusion, a renal diet is a specialized eating plan that supports kidney health and helps people with kidney disease manage their condition. The particular nourishing rules for a renal eating routine spotlight on overseeing protein, sodium, phosph diet to keep up with ideal kidney capability and generally speaking wellbeing. These guidelines concern fluid balance in addition to potassium intake. Managing protein, sodium, potassium, and phosphorus intake is essential for people with renal disease to prevent further damage by limiting protein, sodium, and potassium intake while maintaining adequate fluid intake. By checking these supplements and going with cautious food decisions, people can successfully uphold their kidney wellbeing and work on their personal satisfaction to the kidneys and keep up with in general wellbeing. When developing an individual renal diet plan, it is essential to collaborate closely with a registered dietitian or healthcare professional. A renal diet is specifically designed to help people with kidney disease maintain optimal health by managing their nutrient intake. It is important for people on a renal diet to work closely with a registered dietitian or other healthcare professional to ensure that they are meeting their nutritional needs while adhering to specific to the nutritional needs and goals necessary dietary restrictions. Protein consumption guidelines and restrictions are essential to a renal diet. Protein is a nutrient that the body needs to build and repair tissues. However, consuming an excessive amount of protein can strain the kidneys, particularly in people with kidney disease. In order to avoid further kidney damage, renal diet adherents typically receive advice to cut back on protein consumption. The suggested protein admission for most people with kidney sickness is around 0.6-0.8 grams per kilogram of body weight each day.

People who eat a renal diet need to watch their sodium intake as well as their protein intake. Sodium is a mineral that, when consumed in overabundance, can prompt liquid maintenance and hypertension, which are impeding to kidney wellbeing. As a result, people on a renal diet should limit their sodium intake to less than 2,000 milligrams per day. This can be accomplished by substituting fresh, whole foods for processed and packaged foods, which typically contain a lot of sodium.

CHAPTER44

Food to e avoided for   renal diets

One more significant part of a renal eating regimen is the limitation and suggested consumption for potassium and phosphorus. Mineral called potassium is necessary for a number of bodily functions, including sustaining a healthy heartbeat. However, high blood potassium levels can be dangerous for people with kidney disease. As a result, limiting potassium intake by avoiding foods high in potassium like bananas, oranges, potatoes, and tomatoes is essential. Phosphorus, on the other hand, is a mineral that aids in the development of healthy teeth and bones. Be that as it may, people with kidney illness frequently experience difficulty discharging overabundance phosphorus, prompting significant levels in the blood. Dairy products, nuts, and seeds, among other high-phosphorus foods, should be limited or avoided in order to manage phosphorus intake.

Restrictions and recommended protein, sodium, potassium, and phosphorus intake are all part of a renal diet. By getting it and complying with these rules, people with kidney sickness can more readily deal with their condition and keep up with ideal wellbeing. When developing a bespoke meal plan that is tailored to a person's particular dietary requirements and preferences, it is essential to collaborate closely with a healthcare professional or registered dietitian who specializes in renal nutrition. In addition, individuals on a renal diet may need to make dietary adjustments and regular blood level checks to ensure the best possible outcomes.

Dialysis patients and people with kidney disease can benefit from a renal diet. By limiting one's intake of certain nutrients, such as sodium, potassium, and phosphorus, it aims to ease the burden on the kidneys. Dinner arranging assumes a pivotal part in dealing with a renal eating routine successfully. In order to maintain a balance between meeting nutritional requirements and preventing further kidney damage, it requires careful food selection and portion control.

It is essential to take into account the individual's dietary preferences and restrictions when preparing meals for a renal diet. A renal diet that is well-balanced should include grains, fruits, vegetables, proteins, dairy products, and other foods from different food groups. On the other hand, certain foods should be restricted or avoided entirely. Fast food, processed meats, canned soups, and other foods high in sodium should be avoided as they can raise blood pressure and cause fluid retention. Bananas, oranges, tomatoes, and other potassium-rich foods should also be avoided because they can upset the body's electrolyte balance. All things considered, people can pick lower-potassium choices like apples, berries, and green beans.

First and foremost, limiting sodium intake is essential. Sodium can raise blood pressure and make fluid retention worse, both of which can make the kidneys work harder. As a result, people with kidney disease should try to cut back on the amount of sodium they consume by avoiding processed and packaged foods, which typically contain a lot of sodium. Instead, they ought to select whole, fresh foods and flavor their meals with spices and herbs

Second, people who have kidney disease should watch how much potassium they eat. Elevated degrees of potassium can be unsafe to the heart and can prompt muscle shortcoming and unpredictable heart rhythms. As a result, it's critical to cut back on foods high in potassium like potatoes, bananas, oranges, and tomatoes. All things considered, people can consolidate lower-potassium options like apples, berries, and green beans into their eating regimen.

Lastly, renal diets should control phosphorus as another nutrient. Elevated degrees of phosphorus can prompt bone and heart issues. People with kidney disease should avoid dairy products, nuts, seeds, and processed foods because they contain a lot of phosphorus and can be difficult to control. Before cooking with canned beans, they can also choose to soak and drain them to reduce their phosphorus content.

CHAPTER5

Meal plan nutrition. And Portion control. Of a renal diets

In addition, portion control is essential in a renal diet because it helps control the amount of nutrients that must be consumed. Estimating bits and utilizing more modest plates can be useful in keeping up with the suitable serving sizes. Additionally, people should watch how much fluid they consume because drinking too much fluid can put pressure on the kidneys. It is suggested that people keep track of how much fluid they drink and talk to a doctor about how much fluid is right for their needs and condition. To effectively manage kidney disease and ensure optimal kidney health, a renal diet must include meal planning and portion control.

A renal eating routine, otherwise called a kidney-accommodating eating regimen, is a particular eating plan intended to advance kidney wellbeing and deal with the side effects of kidney sickness. The kidneys assume an imperative part in sifting waste and overabundance liquid from the blood, and when they are not working as expected, certain dietary changes should be made to forestall further harm. A renal diet typically focuses on ensuring adequate protein and other essential nutrients while limiting certain nutrients like sodium, potassium, and phosphorus.

For those who already have kidney disease or are at risk of developing it, understanding renal diets and kidney health is essential. The kidneys are liable for keeping an equilibrium of electrolytes, managing pulse, and sifting byproducts from the body. At the point when kidney capability declines, it can prompt a development of waste and liquid in the body, bringing about different entanglements. People can help slow down the progression of kidney disease, manage symptoms like high blood pressure and fluid retention, and lower their risk of further complications by following a renal diet.

A vital part of a renal eating routine is the limitation of specific supplements that can overwhelm the kidneys. Sodium, for instance, is usually confined in a renal eating routine to assist with controlling circulatory strain and keep up with liquid equilibrium. Potassium and phosphorus are likewise restricted, as elevated degrees of these minerals can be unsafe to people with kidney sickness. On the other hand, protein consumption is typically controlled because too much protein can force the kidneys to work harder. A balanced diet that supports overall health typically includes sources of high-quality protein and other essential nutrients.

In general, knowing about kidney diets and kidney health is important for people with kidney disease or trying to prevent it. Individuals can improve kidney health, manage symptoms of kidney disease, and lower their risk of further complications by adhering to a renal diet. In order to create a bespoke renal diet plan that takes into account each person's requirements, preferences, and stage of kidney disease, it is essential to collaborate closely with a healthcare professional or registered dietitian. By making dietary changes and remaining informed, people can assume command over their kidney wellbeing and further develop their general prosperity.

Dinner making arrangements for a renal eating

routine is significant for people with kidney illness. A renal diet's primary objective is to limit one's intake of certain nutrients, like sodium, potassium, and phosphorus, in order to support optimal kidney function. With regards to dinner anticipating a renal eating regimen, there are a few critical variables to consider.

In conclusion, meal planning for a renal diet is necessary for people with kidney disease to keep their kidneys functioning at their best. People can effectively manage their condition and lessen the strain on their kidneys by controlling their sodium, potassium, and phosphorus intake. Fresh, whole foods should come first, and sodium-laden packaged and processed foods should be avoided. Also, people ought to be aware of their potassium and phosphorus admission and pick lower-potassium and lower-phosphorus options while arranging their feasts.

A special eating plan called a renal diet is meant to help people with kidney disease or other conditions related to the kidney manage their symptoms and avoid further damage to their kidneys. Meal planning is an important part of a renal diet. Meal planning involves choosing and cooking foods low in sodium, potassium, and phosphorus with care.

. Planning your meals is an important part of eating well for your kidneys. There are a few important things to keep in mind when grocery shopping for a renal diet. First and foremost, it is essential to concentrate on whole, fresh foods. Fruits, vegetables, lean proteins, and whole grains must take precedence in this regard. These foods typically contain less sodium and phosphorus, two nutrients that a renal diet must restrict.

Furthermore, it is essential to peruse food names cautiously. Products with low sodium or phosphorus levels should be avoided, as should those with potassium chloride or sodium phosphate.

CHAPTER6

What are the renal diet recipes

By following a renal eating regimen and consolidating recipe thoughts explicitly custom fitted for this eating plan, people can keep up with better command over their kidney wellbeing and further develop their general prosperity.

There are many options for renal diet recipe ideas that can be both nutritious and delicious. A grilled chicken salad with mixed greens, cherry tomatoes, cucumber, and a light vinaigrette dressing is one popular option.

This salad is low in sodium and phosphorus, making it a reasonable choice for those following a renal eating regimen. A salmon fillet baked with lemon and herbs and served with quinoa and steamed asparagus is another recipe idea. Asparagus and quinoa are low in potassium and phosphorus, making this dish kidney-friendly, and salmon is a great source of protein and healthy fats.

Notwithstanding these recipe thoughts, people on a renal eating routine can likewise partake in different soups and stews. A hearty and nutritious option, for instance, is a vegetable and white bean soup made with low-sodium broth, white beans, carrots, celery, and herbs. This soup is low in sodium and potassium while also being high in vitamins and fiber. A chicken and vegetable stew with potatoes, carrots, and green beans is another option. This stew can be a tasty and kidney-friendly dish by using low-sodium broth and reducing the amount of salt added.

CHAPTER 7

What are the feast arrangements for a renal eating routine

In general, feast making arrangements for a renal eating routine is fundamental for people with kidney sickness or other kidney-related conditions. By consolidating recipe thoughts that are low in sodium, potassium, and phosphorus, people can partake in a wide assortment of tasty and nutritious dinners while as yet dealing with their kidneys. It is essential to talk with a medical care proficient or an enrolled dietitian to make a customized feast plan that meets individual dietary requirements and limitations.

Overseeing liquid admission is an Managing fundamental liquid perspective admission is a fundamental of a renal eating routine viewpoint. The kidneys are an important part of a healthy diet, especially for people who have trouble filtering waste kidney and excess disease fluid or who have poor kidney function. the body. At the point when the kidneys are not working as expected The kidneys, liquid play an admission urgent job must in keeping up with the be body's liquid equilibrium cautiously by figured out how to forestall separating liquid over-burden side-effects and keep up with abundance liquid equilibrium from. the bloodstream here is. especially Anyway significant, when for people with ongoing the kidneys kidney are not capability diseaseing appropriately (, they can battle to wipe out overabundance fluid,CKD) or end-stage renal driving illness (toESRD). Liquid maintenance admission and the executives is urgent in forestalling confusions possible such difficulties as. As a result, understanding high blood pressure and the significance of fluid intake and electrolyte management is essential. In this way a renal, understanding the importance dieted of liquid admission.

CHAPTER8

The Management practices in a renal diet

Management in a renal diet is one of the main reasons that people with kidney disease need to control their fluid intake in a renal diet.

One of the main reasons to avoid drinking too much fluid. When the kidneys are unable to manage the condition, a renal diet is essential to effectively reduce excess fluid and prevent fluid overload. When the kidneys aren't working properly, edema occurs when excessive fluid builds up in various parts of the body, such as the legs, ankles, or other areas of swelling. hands. This might liquid reason uneasiness at any point over-burden can contribute and trouble to in breathing high blood. pressure and By observing and strain restricting on liquid admission the, heart people with, potential kidney diseasely prompting could heart at any point forestall liquid disappointment. over-burden and keep a sound By manag fluiding liquid admission balance, people can assist with forestalling these entanglements and in the body.

Another keep a motivation behind why sounds liquid equilibrium consumption.

Moreover the executives are, significant in overseeing liquid admission a renal is diet is crucial for to keeping up with electroly control circulatory strain. The body's blood pressure is high. is electrolyte a common cause of kidney complications like sodium disease, and potassium can further harm the kidneys' calcium. Limit play criticaling jobs liquid in consumption different assists with decreasing the volume of liquid in the substantial body, what capability ins, including muscle turn and assists nerve with working. lower blood pressure when fluid intake is not adequately controlled. can By disturb manag thing liquid equilibrium consumption, of electrolytes people with, kidney sickness can prompting better lopsided characteristics control their that blood can have pressure and unfavorable decrease impacts the on wellbeing risk. For instance, more damage to the kidney. Liquid intake In expansion to can forestalling liquid over-burden andante electrolyte fixations, while deficient liquid admission can controlling blood lead to pressure, overseeing liquid admission in a renal electrolyte uneven characters. Therefore, maintaining management and maintaining electrolyte balance require adequate fluid intake. The overall well-being and electrolyte balance of the kidneys are maintained by this. Role

In conclusion, understanding the significance of sodium, potassium, and phosphorus management in a renal diet in regulating electrolyte levels is essential. When the for people with kidney sickness or kidneys impeded kidney are not capability. working By appropriately, controlling liquid electrolyte consumption, lopsided characteristics people can forestall happen liquid, driving over-burden, to keep a sound different complexities. liquid By balance, cautiously and observing liquid stay away from admission intricacies and such confining as liquids ed asema required and, high blood people with kidney infection can assist with keeping up with legitimate electrolyte pressure. Additionally, managing fluid balance and consuming it reduces complications and the risk of maintaining electrolyte balance.

Finalizing by guaranteeing optimal bodily functions. A focus on monitoring is of the utmost importance in renal diet management and diet regulation. fluid By consuming fluid and comprehending the support significance of kidney health fluid and consuming overall manageme well-being. people with kidney sickness can forestall liquid over-burden, control pulse, and keep up with electrolyte balance. Complying with a renal eating routine that incorporates proper liquid admission rules can enormously work on the personal satisfaction for people with kidney

infection and assist with
protecting kidney capability

CHAPTER9

Overseeing liquid admission is pivotal for people following a renal eating regimen. Hydration plays a significant role in preventing complications and maintaining kidney health. It is essential for people who have kidney disease to find a balance between drinking enough fluids to stay hydrated and limiting fluid intake to avoid overloading the kidneys. Here are a few hints and proposals for remaining hydrated while following a renal eating regimen.

First and foremost, understanding the suggested liquid admission for people with kidney disease is significant. By and large, the suggested liquid admission might differ relying upon elements like age, orientation, and the phase of kidney sickness. However, a common goal is to drink between 1.5 and 2 liters (or 6 and 8 cups) of fluid each day. However, it is essential to consult a registered dietitian or a healthcare professional to ascertain the individual's fluid requirements

As well as observing liquid admission, there are a few systems to help stay hydrated while following a renal eating regimen. Drinking fluids evenly throughout the day is one effective strategy. This implies staying away from unnecessary liquid admission in a brief period and on second thought spreading it out throughout the day. Drinking limited quantities of liquids much of the time can assist with forestalling drying out without overburdening the kidneys. Furthermore, picking the right liquids can likewise add to hydration. For maintaining hydration, herbal teas, low-sodium broths, and water are good options.

Also, people with kidney disease should be careful where they get their fluids. It is crucial for limit or stay away from drinks that can be drying out or unfavorable to kidney wellbeing. This includes coffee, tea, and some soft drinks that contain a lot of caffeine. These drinks may cause dehydration due to their diuretic effect, which causes more urine to be excreted. Drinks with a lot of sodium should also be avoided as much as possible because they can cause fluid retention and strain on the kidneys. To achieve optimal hydration and kidney health, it is essential to strike a balance between fluid intake and renal diet.

CHAPTER10

What are the Tips for shopping food for a renal eating regimen

One more tip for shopping for food for a renal eating regimen is to be aware of piece sizes. It is critical to control segment sizes of high-protein food varieties like meat, poultry, and fish. It is essential to consume these foods in moderation due to their potential high phosphorus content. When you go shopping, look for smaller cuts of meat or frozen or canned versions that often contain less phosphorus.

Furthermore, it means a lot to focus on serving sizes of bundled food varieties and pre-made dinners, as these can frequently contain stowed away wellsprings of sodium and phosphorus.

Last but not least, before going grocery shopping for a renal diet, it's important to think ahead and make a list. You'll be able to stay focused on buying the right foods and remain organized with this. Make a shopping list based on the meals you've planned for the week. This will help you avoid making impulsive purchases and ensure that you have all the ingredients you need to make meals that are good for your kidneys. Furthermore, consider shopping at nearby ranchers' business sectors or specialty stores that offer a more extensive scope of new and low sodium food varieties. By following these tips, shopping for food for a renal eating routine can be made simpler and more viable in supporting your general wellbeing.

THE END